DASH Diet

A Complete Guide to the Dash Diet for Lowering Blood Pressure and Weight Loss, Including Tips, Recipes, and More!

Table Of Contents

Introduction 1
Chapter 1: Boost your Health with DASH Diet Basics 3
Chapter 2: How You Can Follow the DASH Diet Plan 6
Chapter 3: Lowering your High Blood Pressure with DASH. 10
Chapter 4: Losing your Excess Weight with DASH 15
Chapter 5: Sample Meal Plan and Recipes 20
Chapter 6: Quick Tips on How to Benefit the Most
from DASH 27
Conclusion 34

Introduction

I want to thank you and congratulate you for downloading the book, "DASH Diet".

This book contains helpful information about the DASH diet, what it is and how to use it! Through reading this book, you'll be able to understand DASH better, and will learn all about the DASH diet, such as but not limited to the following:

- Why DASH has been voted the best overall diet for five consecutive years

- The benefits you can enjoy through following the DASH Diet principles whether you have high blood pressure or not

- How you can get started with DASH without the usual resistance in following diet plans, as well as how you can transition gradually to DASH

- The significance of reaching and maintaining a healthy weight to lower or stabilize your high blood pressure, and the proven strategies to use DASH in achieving your goals

- How salt or sodium can trigger the rise in your blood pressure and make you carry excess weight, and how DASH can help you lower your sodium consumption and stay within limits

- Why it is necessary and important to eat right, and how you can develop healthy dietary habits through DASH

- How you can design a calorie deficit plan to help you reach and maintain a healthy weight necessary to stop and prevent hypertension, as well as to promote your overall health condition

- How to benefit from an increase in your physical activity critical to succeeding with DASH

- Discover the 2-Phase DASH Plan that can reset your body systems to lose weight more effectively and improve your health

- Look into the sample meal plan and recipes to inspire you in preparing your own plan and recipes to benefit from DASH

Plus you'll find quick tips meant to further increase your success with DASH!

This book includes great tips and techniques that will help you to implement the DASH diet to improve your health, lower blood pressure, and lose weight fast!

Thanks again for downloading this book, I hope you enjoy it!

Chapter 1:
Boost your Health with DASH Diet Basics

The first step in improving your health using the DASH Diet is to start with the basics:

- Get to know what the DASH Diet plan is, and the reasons why it has earned the difficult feat of being voted the best overall diet plan for five consecutive years now

- Discover what benefits await you in using the DASH Diet to improve your health condition

- Understand the principles of the DASH Diet to achieve optimal health

What DASH Stands For

DASH is an acronym for Dietary Approaches to Stop Hypertension. It originated from research by health and nutrition experts for a plan that would lower high blood pressure or hypertension. The US Department of Health and Human Services through the National Institutes of Health (NIH) has sponsored this research.

While the original purpose was to develop a diet plan to stop hypertension, DASH has proven to address other health issues such as diabetes, obesity (excess weight), heart disease and stroke, as well as certain types of cancer. In fact, the U.S. News & World Report has ranked DASH as the best overall diet from 2011 to present.

Results of the original research have paved the way for further studies meant to optimize the diet plan. Thus, from among the diet plans rated by the reputable institution for rankings and advice, the DASH proves to be the best plan for practically everyone who wishes to address health issues, or simply enjoy optimal health.

The Benefits You Get to Enjoy

Most have come to recognize the DASH as the diet that can help address all diseases. All you need to do is to make a few simple changes in your diet and lifestyle, and you are set to enjoy the following:

- Stabilized blood pressure

- Minimized risks of cardiovascular diseases as well as certain cancer types

- A simpler and more effective way to help treat or manage your high blood sugar

- Nutritionally complete diet

- Short-term and long-term weight loss results

- Safest and one of the easiest ways to benefit from following a dietary plan

DASH Diet Principles

The main principle of DASH is to simply improve your eating habits. This allows you to achieve a healthy weight which will in turn lower your blood pressure. Maintaining a healthy weight through eating right will also address health issues other than hypertension.

DASH also emphasizes the importance and necessity of eating vegetables, fruits, and low-fat dairies, as well as whole grains, lean meat, nuts, seeds, and healthy oils. The diet plan also requires you to limit your sodium/salt intake.

Through the DASH Diet plan, you will be able to address nutritional deficiencies found in the standard American Diet. These deficient nutrients are calcium, fiber, magnesium, potassium, and protein. Additionally, by lowering your consumption of sodium/salt and by eating right, you can stop and prevent high blood pressure, maintain a healthy weight, avoid other illnesses, and enjoy an optimal health condition.

Chapter 2:
How You Can Follow the DASH Diet Plan

Expert reviews point to the DASH Diet plan as one of the easiest to follow. Unlike most plans, there are minimal restrictions with DASH. The only strict requirement is for you to limit your sodium/salt intake and to avoid unhealthy food, as much as possible.

What your Plate should Contain

Vegetables, whole grains, and protein should make up your meal plate. The following rules should apply:

- ½ of your plate should consist mostly of vegetables, then fruits, and just the right amount of healthy fats

- ¼ of your plate goes to your protein, and moderate amount of nuts and seeds including legumes

- ¼ of your plate should comprise of your whole grains and low-fat dairy products

Highly flexible, you can customize your meal to adapt to your preferred taste, favorite foods, and routine. This is perhaps the reason why DASH is suitable for practically anyone who wishes to improve his or her health condition.

In brief, here's the foundation for planning your meals under DASH:

Food Type	Servings Per Day	Significance
Vegetables	Minimum of three and up to six servings	Excellent source of fiber, magnesium, and potassium
Fruits	Minimum of four and up to six servings	Essential source of fiber, magnesium, and potassium
Whole Grains	At least six and up to 11 servings	Major source of fiber and energy
Lean meat, fish, and poultry	At least three and maximum of six servings	Main source of protein and magnesium
Fat-free or low-fat dairy products	Two to three servings	Primary source of calcium and protein
Healthy fats and oils	Two to three servings	Important source of calories that also improve the absorption of fat-soluble nutrients

Nuts, Seeds, and Legumes	Three to five servings per week	Rich sources of fiber, protein, energy, and magnesium
Added sugar and low-fat sweets	Two/week to a maximum of five servings per week	In the right amount, sugar or low-fat sweets contribute to taste, and as a carbohydrate, it helps provide energy and food for the brain.

The DASH Eating Plan Chart includes some additional details that you can use to plan your meals.

Gradual Transition

The way to succeed in following DASH is to make a gradual transition from your existing diet, especially if you are used to the American Diet. Transitioning slowly but surely will minimize the pressure and resistance.

It's pleasantly surprising that you can also observe the DASH principles when you dine out. Solutions are handy owing to the flexibility of the diet plan and the minimal restrictions it carries.

Here's a recommended 3-step strategy to guarantee success in transitioning to the DASH Diet Plan:

1. Write the changes you wish to make in your diet to follow DASH

2. Check if these changes are S-M-A-R-T (specific, measureable, attainable, realistic and relevant, and track-able)

3. Start making the changes one change at a time

DASH is easy to follow as there is not much restriction. It is important, though, to eat right and choose foods rich in nutrients to resolve your health issue/s and to stay healthy. You can never go wrong with eating vegetables and fruits and choosing whole-foods over processed foods.

Chapter 3:
Lowering your High Blood Pressure with DASH

The most effective natural method to stop and prevent high blood pressure is to eat healthily. Perhaps, the best way to do this is through DASH. You'll find out how with the strategies you'll discover here.

Reach and Maintain your Healthy Weight

Several studies have established the relationship between one's body weight and blood pressure regardless of age. Results have shown that losing excess weight, especially when one is obese, lowers blood pressure. Excess body weight triggers the blood pressure to rise.

If you are suffering from hypertension, chances are great that you carry excess weight. Thus, losing weight is one of the first things you need to do to normalize your blood pressure. If you don't have hypertension, you will still benefit a lot from maintaining a healthy weight.

How do you know that you are at your healthy weight? The WebMD recommends two things to measure: (1) body mass index or BMI and (2) waist circumference.

To calculate your BMI, you may want to use the tool provided by the NHI. You just have to know your height and weight and enter the digits. If your BMI is:

- Less than 18.5, you are underweight

- Between 18.5 – 24.9, you are in your normal weight

- In the range of 25-25.9, you are overweight

- 30 or greater means that you have obesity

However, BMI is just one of the two factors to determine healthy weight. It may not always be totally accurate. If you carry a lot of muscle, you may be healthy, however the BMI total will say that you are overweight/obese, so keep this in mind when testing yourself.

A great way to determine if you should lose weight is to pay attention to how your waist measures. Fat in your abdominal area causes a higher risk of heart disease and other weight-related health conditions such as hypertension.

Measure your waist and see if you fall under any of these digits that represent healthy waist size:

- For men, your waist size should measure 40-36 inches or less (102-91 cm)

- For women, your waist size should measure 35-32 inches or less (88-81 cm)

To lose excess weight, start changing your dietary habits. Shift to DASH to achieve your healthy weight. You will be able to either lower your high blood pressure if you are already hypertensive, or maintain your healthy weight to prevent hypertension.

How DASH can Help you Reach a Healthy Weight

DASH encourages you to develop healthy eating habits. You will learn how to eat right when you transition to this diet plan. It can bring both short-term and long-term weight loss.

It is as simple as increasing your intake of vegetables, fruits and whole grains and choosing real food over processed food.

Here are some techniques you can use to help you achieve and maintain your healthy weight with DASH:

- Learn how to benefit from healthy substitution. For instance, instead of enjoying your usual potato chips, substitute them with baked or boiled sweet potato. Why snack with junk when you can choose a serving of fresh fruit and vegetables that provide way more energy?

- To increase your consumption of vegetables, mix it with your favorite food. For instance, if you love eating hamburgers, decrease the amount of lean meat and then add vegetables such as carrots, onions, kale or spinach as substitute.

- Follow the recommended serving sizes. You do not have to eat only vegetables and fruits, but you can actually eat various food types within their daily serving sizes. Use the <u>DASH Eating Plan Chart</u> as your guide.

Do More Physical Activity

Part of DASH is to increase your physical activities. This does not only help you stop and prevent hypertension, but it also minimizes your risks of heart attack and stroke.

You only need to allot 30 minutes a day on most days during the week to do moderate physical activity. Examples are the following:

- Wash your car or your windows/floor for 45 minutes to an hour

- Walk the stairs for about 15 minutes

- Play volleyball for about an hour, or basketball for about 30 minutes

- Dancing for about 30 minutes

- Do water aerobics for about 30 minutes

- Jump rope for 15 minutes

- Running for at least one (1) mile in 10 minutes

If your chosen activity requires 30 minutes, you don't even have to consume all 30 minutes straight! You can divide it into three sessions of 10 minutes each or two sessions of 15 minutes each as well as 20 and 10 minutes each.

Note, however, that if you have an existing health condition, it is prudent to consult your physician prior to increasing your physical activity, especially if this is the first time you will be doing moderate physical activity.

Decrease your Intake of Sodium

If there is one requirement or restriction that DASH is strict about, it is the consumption of sodium or salt. DASH recommends that you consume food types that are low in sodium, so you can keep up with the requirement of between 2,300 mg/day to 1,500 mg/day.

Why You Have to Limit your Sodium Intake

Excess sodium in the body puts pressure on your heart and your blood vessels. This triggers your blood pressure to rise in a condition you know as hypertension or high blood pressure.

This is because sodium or salt encourages your body to retain water that in turn interferes with the normal functions of your heart and blood vessels.

DASH restricts your daily consumption to 2,300 mg/day or about one (1) teaspoon of salt, or preferably 1,500 mg/day or about ¾ teaspoon of salt per day. Note that most foods contain sodium, even those that do not taste salty.

Processed, fast, and instant food items are the types that are rich in sodium. Thus, you are better off choosing whole or real foods just as DASH would recommend. Further, instead of using salt to add flavor and taste to your dishes, use spices such as pepper among others.

Chapter 4:
Losing your Excess Weight with DASH

You have learned from the previous chapter that reaching a healthy weight is one of the most effective ways to stop and prevent hypertension. Whether or not you are hypertensive, you can benefit vastly from DASH in getting rid of your excess weight. Here's how to do it.

Choose to Eat Right

DASH gives you the freedom to choose the food that you eat. Thus, if you wish to lose your excess weight, choose to eat right. Eating right means focusing on food types that are high in nutrients, especially foods that will allow you to correct the nutritional deficiencies found in the standard American diet.

It also means eating various food types in their recommended serving sizes, and be sure to follow the restriction or limit on sodium consumption. If you have to use or consume packaged food or ingredients, it pays to read the "Nutrition Facts" label to check for sodium content.

While salt and sodium are interchangeable, they are two different things. Salt or sodium chloride preserves and flavors food. Sodium, meanwhile, is one of the elements that make up salt. Common food additives usually contain sodium such as baking soda, MSG, and sodium nitrite.

Design a Calorie Deficit Plan

To lose weight, you can design your own calorie deficit plan using the DASH principles. Calorie deficit means that the calories that you consume should be less than the calories that you expend. Your diet should allow your body to burn more calories than what it receives. However, this should not mean compromising your nutritional requirements.

Hence, the DASH serves this purpose well since it allows you to receive the nutrients your body needs from all food groups. To design your calorie deficit plan, use the following steps:

- Determine your healthy weight (as discussed in the previous chapter), and then set your weekly weight loss goal. Start with a ½ pound of weight loss target for the week, then gradually increase your target but do not exceed 2 pounds of weight loss per week.

- Find out your calorie requirements. The requirements depend on your gender (male, female) your age, as well as the level of your physical activity. The chart below, taken from the NIH site, illustrates the daily calorie requirements. When you have calculated your daily energy expenditure, aim for a 200-500 calorie deficit per day. Keep in mind that the figures in the below chart are estimates, and will vary depending on your size, body composition, and metabolism. Weigh yourself at the start of the week, stick to a calorie deficit, and then weigh yourself at the end. This will help you to gauge if you are eating a sufficient amount, not enough, or too much.

Your Daily Calorie Needs

Gender	Age (years)	Calories Needed for Each Activity Level		
		Sedentary	Moderately Active	Active
Female	19–30	2,000	2,000–2,200	2,400
	31–50	1,800	2,000	2,200
	51+	1,600	1,800	2,000–2,200
Male	19–30	2,400	2,600–2,800	3,000
	31–50	2,200	2,400–2,600	2,800–3,000
	51+	2,000	2,200–2,400	2,400–2,800

- Choose from the DASH Eating Plan Chart how to meet your calorie requirements. This will help you get rid of your excess weight without compromising your nutritional requirements. Chances are that your calorie intake is greater than what your body actually needs. Following the chart allows you to lower your caloric intake, but not to the point of nutritional deficiency.

Increase your Physical Activity

The best results of weight loss come when you combine DASH with moderate physical activities that you do regularly. To lose weight effectively, the surest way is to lower your calorie consumption, and at the same time increase your physical activity.

Here are some examples of moderate physical activity from the Harvard School of Public Health:

- Brisk walking of 4 miles per hour

- Mop the floor or wash your windows

- Play badminton or tennis

With moderate physical activity, you'll be able to burn more calories - up to six (6) times more per minute compared to sedentary activity. It is also through your physical activity that you'll be able to sustain and maintain your weight loss results from DASH.

Use the 2-Phase Plan as a Guide

Marla Heller of "The DASH Diet Weight Loss Solution" who is a registered dietician recommends the two-phase plan for weight loss:

- Phase 1 is where you are going to get rid of your excess weight, especially around your waistline. This will let you achieve a healthy weight. During this phase, you will train your body to respond only to real hunger. You will have to avoid foods with sugar and starches including fruits and whole grains. This phase lasts 14 days or two (2) weeks.

- Phase 2 is where you will reintroduce fruits and whole grains and eat healthy foods from the <u>DASH Eating Plan Chart.</u> It is during this phase that you will maintain your weight loss results; hence, it has no duration and you can continue with this phase as long as you wish to stay within your healthy weight. Your weight loss results should continue throughout this phase, but may be stopped once you reach your ideal target weight.

You can customize this weight loss solution to suit your specific needs, just keep the basics in mind. An example of this is the 7-Day DASH diet meal plan published at the official website of Dr. Oz.

Chapter 5:
Sample Meal Plan and Recipes

Create a DASH meal plan that you'll be able to follow consistently. You can choose to create a daily planner or a weekly planner depending on your preference and convenience. DASH is highly flexible and customizable, and as such, you can surely make it work to your success!

Sample Meal Plan

Here's an example of DASH Meal Plan:

Calorie Needs	Meal	Food & Serving Size
2,000 calories	Breakfast	Two servings of cooked oatmeal One cup of milk 1 medium-sized apple One slice of whole wheat bread Two tablespoons of peanut butter
	Lunch	Mixed vegetable salad One to two cups of strawberry-lemon juice A cup of fruit medley
	Snacks	A cup of Greek yogurt with banana slices 1/3 cup of roasted and unsalted almonds

	Dinner	A cup of brown rice Up to two servings of roasted chicken breast Half a cup of green veggies Up to two servings of your preferred seasonal fruit
1,600 calories	Breakfast	A slice of whole wheat bread One tablespoons of peanut butter A cup of skimmed milk A cup of melons
	Lunch	Chicken Caesar sandwich A cup of corn and carrots 1 medium-sized banana One cup of vegetable juice
	Snacks	You may choose to skip or snack on nuts, but only thrice per week and limit your serving to 1/3 cup, you may also enjoy ½ cup of fresh fruit juice such as lemonade
	Dinner	Roast beef salad A cup of green beans One piece of small apple

		A cup of low fat to nonfat milk
	Lunch	Chicken breast salad 2 slices of toasted whole wheat bread Up to teaspoons of soft margarine A 4 oz. glass of grapefruit drink I medium-sized apple
	Snacks	A cup of nonfat fruit yogurt Half a cup of frozen berries A cup of sliced cucumbers Up to 14 pieces of carrot sticks
	Dinner	One cup of spaghetti or tuna pesto Mixed green salad A cup of mixed fresh fruits A cup of apple juice
2,600 calories	Breakfast	One cup of bran cereals One cup low fat milk One medium banana Up to two slices of whole wheat bread One teaspoon butter or soft margarine A cup of orange juice

Lunch		Chicken breast salad
		2 slices of toasted whole wheat bread
		Up to teaspoons of soft margarine
		A 4 oz. glass of grapefruit drink
		I medium-sized apple
Snacks		A cup of nonfat fruit yogurt
		Half a cup of frozen berries
		A cup of sliced cucumbers
		Up to 14 pieces of carrot sticks
Dinner		One cup of spaghetti or tuna pesto
		Mixed green salad
		A cup of mixed fresh fruits
		A cup of apple juice

Sample Recipes

Breakfast

Breakfast Oats	
Ingredients	2 cups of steel cut oats 2 to 3 cups of skimmed or low fat milk 2 teaspoon of vanilla ½ teaspoon of cinnamon powder ¾ cup of sliced banana
Procedure	1. Cook the oatmeal according to package instruction. 2. Adjust your stove to low heat, and then add the skimmed milk, vanilla, and cinnamon powder. Mix. 3. Add the banana slices and continue to simmer for two minutes.

Lunch

Chicken Caesar Sandwich

Ingredients	One boneless chicken breast Romaine lettuce One medium-sized white onion One piece of tomato One piece cucumber 2 cloves of garlic, minced 2 tablespoons of Caesar salad dressing 1 tablespoon of olive oil 1 tablespoon of grated natural cheddar cheese Pepper to taste 2 slices of whole wheat bread

Snacks

Berry Yogurt

Ingredients	One cup of mixed berries 2 cups of low fat Greek yogurt Up to two teaspoons of raw honey 2 tablespoons of toasted crushed almonds
Procedure	1. Combine the first two ingredients. 2. Top with raw honey and toasted almonds.

Dinner

Hot Tuna Pesto Salad

Ingredients	Canned hot tuna in water, drained (or find one that contains minimal salt/sodium) Pesto (you can make your own or buy commercially available mix) Spinach Fettuccine One tablespoon of olive oil ¼ cup of sliced black olives A teaspoon of oregano Medium-sized white onion, chopped 2 cloves of garlic, minced 1 teaspoon of unsalted butter Pepper to taste
Procedure	1. Cook your fettuccine following package instruction. 2. In a saucepan, sauté your butter, garlic, and onion. 3. When the garlic starts to brown and the onion becomes translucent, add your tuna and pepper. 4. Mix well, and then add the oregano. 5. Continue mixing while adding the pesto. 6. When the mixture is ready, combine it with your pasta. 7. Drizzle with olive oil.

Chapter 6:
Quick Tips on How to Benefit the Most from DASH

Prevent Hypertension Before It Happens

It is always best to prevent high blood pressure before it happens. Thus, whether or not you are hypertensive, start the transition to DASH that will enable you to:

- Consume just the right amount of saturated fat as well as cholesterol

- Increase your consumption of foods rich in calcium, potassium, fiber, and magnesium, as well as protein, and nutrients that help stabilize your blood pressure.

- Meet your nutritional requirements while decreasing your salt consumption.

Make it a habit to:

- Check your blood pressure, especially if risk factors are present. A normal blood pressure measures at <120 / <80. Any value higher puts you at risk of hypertension. If your blood pressure measures at 140 or above/90 or above, you are classified as having hypertension.

- Eat healthily. Understand that any rise in your blood pressure can bring serious health risks. Thus, be sure to take the necessary steps in stabilizing your blood pressure within normal levels. Remember that prevention is much better than a cure.

- Follow the <u>DASH Eating Plan Chart.</u> This tip is worth repeating since when you master the chart and recognize its importance, everything else will be a breeze. They key is to acquire the habit of eating right and when you do, you will no longer have to worry about your blood pressure.

Lose Weight without Even Trying

Think of weight loss as a side effect of DASH. In developing healthy dietary habits through DASH and by lowering your intake of sodium/salt, you can lose weight minus the typical ordeals involved. All you need to get rid of your excess weight is to eat right, which you can develop through DASH.

Keep these in mind:

- Most of the salt or sodium that we consume comes from processed food, instant food, and fast food. Sodium is typically present in the following food: baked goods and pastries, monosodium glutamate (MSG), junk food, certain cereals, and baking soda.

- Always complete your essential meals for the day, every day: breakfast, lunch, and dinner as well as two (2) to three snacks. Be sure to refer to your <u>DASH Eating Plan Chart</u> or your daily/weekly meal plan. Avoid depriving yourself of your meals, as deprivation can only result in adverse effects.

- Make your vegetables and fruits colorful, as they are rich in nutrients that will help you stop and prevent hypertension, lose excess weight and maintain a healthy weight, and help resolve multiple health issues. See the following table:

Red	Lowers high blood pressure, prevents tumor growth, reduces the risk of prostate cancer, decreases the level of bad cholesterol, and searches for free radicals to prevent damage, helps in the treatment and prevention of arthritis.
Yellow	Prevents degenerative diseases, delays aging, lowers high blood pressure and bad cholesterol, and flushes out toxins in the body.
Orange	Strengthens the immune system, promotes healthy skin and joints, fights free radicals, promotes the good balance of alkaline and acid, and helps in improving bone health.
Green	Builds and promotes healthy cells, discourages and prevents the formation of cancer cells, detoxifies the body, stabilizes blood pressure, keeps bad cholesterol from overpowering good cholesterol, improves digestive health, fights free radicals, and helps to rebuild the immune system.

Blue	Annihilates free radicals, boosts immunity, promotes digestive health, and inhibits cancer cells.
Purple	Promotes good vision and eye health, lowers bad cholesterol, and improves the body's absorption of nutrients. Is also anti-inflammatory, anti-carcinogen.
White	Boosts the immune system, kills cancer cells particularly those that cause breast, colon, and prostate cancers, promotes the good balance of hormones, lowers the risks of hormonal diseases and endocrine disorders.

Make your Physical Activity your Healthy Habit

To succeed with DASH is not just about eating right. It is also about developing the healthy habit of exercising or increasing your physical activity. Most people find it difficult to maintain an exercise routine or to increase their physical activity, but this difficulty disappears once they have formed the habit.

You may want to consider the following:

- Choose to increase an activity that you are already doing, e.g. house chores. For instance, instead of washing your floor once a month, do it twice a month initially and then once every week.

- Choose an activity that can fit into your schedule easily, so that you can't use your schedule as an excuse. Perhaps, amongst all, walking is the most flexible activity that you can do on a regular basis.

- Choose an activity that you love or enjoy doing. This way, there will be minimal resistance, if any. Doing something that you love or enjoy will make you look forward to doing it repeatedly until it becomes your habit. An example would be joining a sporting team.

There is no way around it. To speed up the weight loss process, improve your health, and make exercise a habit, you must do the following:

| Start the Routine | Create Your Schedule | Do It Repeatedly |

- In starting an exercise routine, do it at the same time and place as much as possible. This will make it easier for you to repeat the activity and form it into your healthy habit.

- Plan and calendar your activity. Scheduling the activity should encourage you to do it without interruptions. Thinking about what you have to do, as scheduled, makes you want to do it more.

- Keep on doing the activity consistently, preferably at the same time and place, for at least three (3) months. In developing the habit, the key is repetition.

Create your Shopping List

To make it convenient and easy for you to eat right, it helps to create your DASH shopping list. Buy only what's on your list when you go to the grocery store, and always consider the DASH Eating Plan Chart when creating your list.

The Mayo Clinic has these tips:

- Refer to your DASH meal plan when you create your shopping list. This way, you'll be able to include all ingredients that you need in preparing your meals for the week.

  The list will prevent you from spending unnecessarily, while also avoiding temptations to stray from your diet plan.

- Observe the cardinal rule in grocery shopping: eat first. This will enable you to resist processed and fast food while shopping for your grocery items.

- Stick to your list. Visit the areas where you can find fresh food, whole food, or real food. As much as possible, avoid or limit going to areas where you can find processed, instant, and junk food items.

- Make it a habit to read the "Nutrition Facts" label. You'll be able to make better choices and stay away from items that have a high sodium content.

- See to it that you buy the following staples: multi-colored vegetables and fruits, whole grains, low fat to nonfat dairy products, lean meat including fish meat and poultry, nuts and seeds including legumes, and spices and herbs as well as condiments (low salt or sodium) to add flavor and taste to your dishes.

Conclusion

Thank you again for downloading this book!

I hope this book was able to help you learn more about the DASH diet! Understanding how the DASH works through the basics provided in this book should help you reach your goals in using the diet plan.

By now, you should be familiar with the following:

- The principles of the DASH Diet, specifically the importance of eating right

- The DASH Eating Plan Chart that lists the food groups, the recommended daily servings and their serving sizes, as well as the significance of including these food items/ingredients in your meals

- How to use your DASH Diet plan to lower or stabilize your blood pressure

- How to lose weight without even trying

- The things you can do to develop the healthy habit of eating right and increasing your physical activity, as well as sticking to your DASH Diet to sustain and maintain your success

The next step is to put the strategies provided into use, and begin implementing the DASH diet yourself! You can do it and earn your success with commitment and discipline.

Finally, if you enjoyed this book, please take the time to share your thoughts and post a review on Amazon. It'd be greatly appreciated!

Thank you and good luck!

www.ingramcontent.com/pod-product-compliance
Lightning Source LLC
LaVergne TN
LVHW021744060526
838200LV00052B/3455